Voices

Jan Hahn M.D.

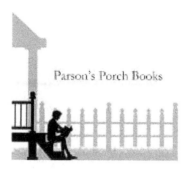

Parson's Porch Books

Voices

ISBN: Softcover 978-1-960326-12-6

Copyright © 2023 by Jan Hahn, M.D.

Parson's Porch Books is an imprint of Parson's Porch *&* Company (PP*&*C) in Cleveland, Tennessee. PP*&*C is a self-funded charity which earns money by publishing books of noted authors, representing all genres. Its face and voice is **David Russell Tullock** (dtullock@parsonsporch.com).

Parson's Porch *&* Company *turns books into bread & milk* by sharing its profits with the poor.

www.parsonsporch.com

Contents

To the Reader

The structure of this work is quite straightforward.

In a sparsely furnished family physician's office, patients arrive alone to tell their story.

What is important to this doctor? Only that which is important to his patients - nothing more and nothing less.

Some come once, never to return. Others frequent his office repeatedly as they struggle to make sense of what has befallen them.

None come for judgment; a few for advice; but all simply to be heard.

On the left facing page are notations of several types:

VOICE OVER - introduces the speaker

&- commentary on how the poem is to be read

&&- personal reflections of the writer on the meaning of the poem

Readers may very well wonder if each poem represents a single patient. In a few instances, this is the case. But most of them are composites based upon repeated contact with people who have contended, in their unique ways, with common crises.

I have been privileged to have had no less than 150,000 patient encounters (100 patients per week - 50 weeks per year - 30 years).

Despite our differences, at the end of the day, we confront the same basic issues of life and living.

Appearances

Beneath the mirror surface of the placid sea,
Roll waves too fierce to safely plumb.

Thus, doth calm countenance masks a troubled heart
And cheerful mien, a wounded soul.

Voice Over

"Rose - what brings us together today?"

❧

She begins very matter-of-factly but quickly anger bubbles to the surface, reaching a crescendo in her caustic put-down of the doctor.

❧❧

What does a person really want from life?

First - that their basic needs be met - food, clothing, and shelter.

Second - that they are not subjected gratuitously to abuse - physical, sexual, or emotional.

Third - that someone, one day, loves them fc

Fourth, but no less important than the other   e
of who they are or what they provide but simply because, in the words of the Bible, they were fashioned in the image of God.

Rose says as much in this bitter accounting of her life.....

Nerves

I was born thirty-five years ago, come September.
Nashville, I believe, or maybe Memphis.
First child of a sixteen-year-old girl and a no-name
Creature of the gutter.
One night stand - don't reckon he is alive anymore.
I got his temper or so my mother says.

By twelve, I had five "fathers" - if that is what you call a man that Screws
your mother.
Two taught me sex their way. (Let's not go there today, Doc.)

Pot, coke, acid - tasted all by sixteen.
What other pleasures are there, when life is only pain?

Left school in tenth
What it taught; I had no use for.
What I needed to know; it could not teach.

I have two sons: Jason from Robert and Eric from Thomas.
Or perhaps it was the other way around.
No matter. Not seen either for years.

I smoke two packs a day and drink only at night.
How else can one sleep and not dream?

Money? Welfare check at the first of the month.
And don't you be running your mouth and telling everybody that I practice The
oldest profession in the world.
It's not hard work - the old ones, like you Doc, peter out pretty fast.

Why am I here today?
I'm nervous dammit. I need a pill.
And I hear you listen.

Voice Over
> *"Mrs. Watson, and what brings us together today?"*

&

This is a woman whose conflicting impulses wage war on her psyche. Torn between the unforgiving dictates of marriage and the pain of rejection, she questions her love. Her actions give no one else cause to doubt; it is her thoughts that frighten her.

&&

One marries and promises to be faithful to the end. But when does the end occur?

Alzheimer's

Sixty years.
Robbed the cradle, that's what they say.
Paw had to sign a note to let me go.

We had nine children - buried two before five - seventeen grandchildren
and three great-grandchildren.

Every night for more than a half century, I slept with him.
We could talk without speaking.

Now, he loses everything. Can't remember names and sometimes forgets
to pull down his drawers. (I wash often.)
Mostly he just sits.
Is he happy?

He pees on the floor - he laughs.
He puts his pants on his head - he laughs.
He throws food at the cat - he laughs.
I suppose so.

Calls me Grace. My name is Ruth Ann. Grace is the girl he was courtin' til I
appeared and stole his heart.

Doc, is it evil to pray for a man's death?

Voice Over
"Mr. Cavanaugh - What can I do for you today?"

Chronic pain saps the will and crushes the spirit. It makes a man bitter and mean. And those who try to help are frequently subjected to the fury of the tortured.

Pain

It's my back.

I can't sleep.
I can't work.
I can't even screw my old lady.

Three oxy's a day is all I need.

Don't give me Prozac.
I'm not depressed - anymore than you would be if
all you could do is sit and shit.

Don't give me mood stabilizers.
I would cry if it wouldn't hurt so much.

Arthritis pills tear up my guts.
Muscle relaxants just make me tired.

How come Joe gets two a day? He have something on you?
I could get all I need off the streets but why make me break the law?

You're a God damn fucking SOB.
What sort of doc are you?
If you can't cure, you could at least care.

Voice Over

"Mr. Wilson - How are you doing today?"

❦

Mr. Wilson is an obnoxious, self-centered man who has an inflated sense of importance. He has little need for the doctor or at least no more use for him than that which he has for his mechanic. And he lets him know that.

❦❦

Wealth and power and the axis of success spins between them.

Busy Man - Part I

I'm a busy man and don't have time for foolishness.
You have one month to control my blood pressure, or I find a doc who
knows what he is doing.

Do you know how much I make?
In three months, I surpass your year.

What do I want in life?
(So you are turning existential on me?)

Money and power.
What else is there worth striving for?

Voice Over

"Lisa, I trust that all is right with you?"

This woman is out of control, careening down a highway at ever increasing speeds. A crash is inevitable but until that moment, Lisa loves every minute of the journey. She overwhelms you, captivating you with her sheer exuberance and lack of restraint. Could we not all be so uninhibited?

Bipolar disorder is one of the most destructive psychiatric conditions. Just ask the many victims who lay by the side of the road.

Bizywoman

Whazzup doc?
How are you doing? Fine? Only fine? I'm great!!

Three jobs now:
Selling jewelry
Flipping burgers
Driving cars
By next month, I'll be manager at all three.

Sleep? Sleep is for sissies but sex isn't.
You look mighty tempting today.
I bet that each morning your wife says you're one hot cookie.
Tell me - do you like her sunnyside up or sunnyside down?
(Doc, I think you're blushing.)
Sex is like food - variety is the spice of life.
So if you want to ever taste a new dish -

Gonna hold off on the medicines this month.
Why? Three reasons:
They're expensive.
They drag me down.
I can't remember to take them anyway.

Gotta go - got people to meet, things to do and places to see.

As the Frenchies say - "Au revoir!"

Voice Over

"Mr. Jeffers, what brings us together today?"

&

Mr. Jeffers reacts with the outraged and anguished cry of a man whose soul has just been impaled. Let no one doubt that the pain is so viscerally perceived that rational thought is impossible.

&&

Infidelity is a crime not only against man but also against God. The fabric of the family is literally shredded by the arrogant selfishness of one spouse. There can be no love where there is no trust. And where there is no love, there is no life worth living.

Trust

My wife has had an affair!

Trust is like the sand dunes on the ocean's shore.
Each grain borne to the water's edge by ceaseless tide, fired by sun,
burnished by wind packs deep and hard.

A testament to the power of time - or so it seems.

But Mother Nature is a fearsome and frightful force, who seizes what she
desires and has no conscience.

And in a day of thoughtless anger or a night of ill-conceived passion, levels all
Leaving no trace of eon's work.

Voice Over

"Debra, how are you today?"

Debra begins as she expects others expect her to. But once she beings to describe her ailment, a pensive - almost frightened - demeanor emerges. The doctor's quiet demonstration of interest and care convinces her to speak the unspeakable.

We watch our children grow up to become young adults full of enthusiasm for a world they have yet to experience. We envy their naivete, enjoy vicariously their adventures and fearfully imagine the worst that can befall them.

Mission Trip

I'm back from my mission trip!
To spread the word of Jesus Christ to those who know nothing of him - is a
blessing few can be privileged to receive.
Glory Glory Glory- his name is one!

Any problems?
Only one for which my mother made me come.
My stomach hurts - actually the site is a little further south (but don't tell my
mother)

For two months I've had a pain.
Sometimes it is a twinge of discomfort - sufficient only to
remind me of its presence.
But then it will explode into my consciousness and
blot out all competing thought.
It comes without warning, lasts seconds or many hours.
Nothing makes it better nor makes it worse.
Nor does any other symptom share its space.

I can tell by your face that you are deeply puzzled and so am I.

Is there anything else I want to say?
Do you have the time?
Of course, you always do.

It was a bright August afternoon and I worked quietly alone in the
schoolhouse-

The children having happily fled hours earlier.
I did not notice two men enter
'til one across my face wrapped his hand
And the other locked the door.

Voice Over

"Mr. Philpot, what brings us together today?"

Confusion, anger and fear – all mixed together in an inchoate stew of emotion.

All of us desperately want to believe there is some ultimate meaning to our existence: that we are more than prairie grace destined only fo a brief moment in the sun. Yet when the evidence is unciakable – for why else would on have survived – and the reason remains obscure – where can the answer be found.

Design or Luck?

Why am I here?
Why do I stand upon this earth and take up space?

Last month, my heart stopped, and I was jolted out of the hands of Death.
I stood at the edge of my grave, then turned and walked away.

God does nothing without reason.
But I'll be damned if I know what he has in store for me.

You're smart! Can you not divine?
Show me your order sheet.
Is there not a test that uncovers meaning or fathoms purpose?

Voice Over

"Mr. Simpson, Good Day."

❧

A bitter angry man whose useful life seems over. Nothing remains but the dreadful task of watching oneself deteriorate while remembering the long-gone pleasures of the past.

❧❧

Where there is no meaning, existence is a struggle. And with each passing day, harder to justify.

Retirement

Hello Doc.
Why am I here?
Because I have nothing better to do.
I retired one year to the day.
And am bored, bored, bored.
Boredom weighs across my shoulders like a yoke across a mule's back.
My yoke is too heavy to bear.
I groan with each step I take.

I have labored all my life.
My father was a farmer.
I roused the rooster, then did the morning chores.
In high school, I worked in a lumber yard.
Do you know how heavy a 2" by 12' plank is?
There was nothing I could not shoulder.

I loved the feel of wood in my coarsened hands and
The sweet smell of freshly cut pine.
So I became a builder- a hundred homes these hands built.
The Preston Place on Deventer Ridge - my hands.
The Stiles home on Kingston Avenue - my hands.
The Oglethorpe mansion - my hands.

Do I enjoy my wife?
Let me tell you about her.
When first we met, God, was she a beauty.
A waist around which I could clasp my two hands,
Breasts and hips that made men ache to touch.
But today, her breasts hang like a pendulum on an old Swiss clock;
Her ass is so big it swallows the chair upon which she sits.
I have no desire for her nor does she me.

These pills you gave me so I could live "a long and healthful life to
enjoy the fruits of my labors" - - -
Take them!
There are no pleasures in my world - the money I spend on medicine,
I would my children have.

Voice Over

"Mr. Broadtree, What is your concern today?"

❧

He speaks with a quiet reminiscent tone, not a trace of bitterness in his voice. But it ends with a note of wistfulness that makes one wonder what will he be thinking.

❧❧

I love to listen to the old relive their past.
One learns lessons on how to live. Today, so many feel entitled to the fruits of their labor without having to labor.

Breakin' Down

It's my blood pressure pills- they're just not workin'.
I think I am getting old and Doc, you seem to be
runnin' out of patches for this
Creakin' collection of bones.
Do you have any bailing wire and duck tape in your bag?

I heard in the news today that scientists have found a potion
to make old rats young again.
Now, would if I could take such a pill?
Not if I had to relive my past.

We were poor folk. Dad was ill and could not work
so when I was six and my sisters eight and ten,
we were hired out to the neighbors.
Every morning we rose at four to milk their cows and gather eggs.
It was so cold in the winter that our clothes soon wet, quickly froze.
Our hands numb from use - our backs aching.
Seven days a week, week after week, month after month, year after year.
The Good Book says that on the seventh day the Lord rested from his labors
and so should man.
But let me tell you this, my friend, cows and chickens
don't read the Good Book.
The eldest drove us mercilessly but every week we brought home $15
And we survived.

When I was eighteen, I got married and became a mechanic.
Never missed a day 'til I retired.
Married my high school sweetheart and have never
cast my eyes upon another woman.
Raised three - now all gone.

I am tired but I'm proud of what I've done and have no regrets.
Would I, if I could take such a pill?
Old men have only memories to keep them company,
Now your question makes me dream.

Voice Over

"Mr. Bolt, We have a lot to talk about today."

&

Even if our rational self knows otherwise, our heart believes in immortality. Mr. Bolt, powerful and always in control, cannot believe the sentence. His outrage shakes the room.

&&

Dr. Kubler-Ross documented the stages a person traverses when he confronts his imminent mortality. This is the first of a series of poems that explores how patients respond to this ultimate challenge.

Cut and Deal

So there is no way to win?
There is no cure for this disease?
Only... what was the word you mumbled? Palliation?
You're a fool.

Do you know who I am?
I command hundreds, spend millions every year and
hobnob with the famous.

I am a lion!
When I roar, the earth trembles.

So here's the deal.

Tell me the cost of the cure, I'll pay it now.
There is no expense I cannot bear.

Voice Over

"Mr. Sanders, It is truly good to see you back."

❦

In a foxhole, there are no atheists. Let Mr. Sanders show you why. His honesty and self-deprecating humor reflect the thoughts of a man who has changed.

❦❦

At the moment when all control must be ceded, to whom does one turn - man or God? Or perhaps both and hedge your bet.

The Operation

How did the operation go?
Well.
Actually, the surgeon said - "Far better than expected."

It's because I prayed.
Don't laugh at me.
I know that once I said,
"Religion is solace for weak-willed frightened souls."
But there are times one must hedge their bets.

"God- I know you are busy.
Please - a moment of your time.
My friends and family ask me: How do I feel?
Fine is my reply.
But between you and me,
I'm fuckin' scared.

God - I know you are busy,
But tomorrow, hold tight the surgeon's hand."

Voice Over

"Melinda, Hello my friend, can we talk?"

Anger smolders beneath the surface in this young lady then erupts like a flame engulfing a house. She cries out for help even as she rejects its offer.

Anorexia nervosa has a significant mortality rate. And it inflicts its toll disproportionately upon very bright upper middle-class white women. In a society whose population is growing increasingly obese yet remains obsessed about thinness, anorexia nervosa seems nothing less than a horrible curse meant to mock us.

Weight

I understand, Doc, about my weight you wish to talk
5'4" and 90 pounds

Is that your concern?

I am a puppet upon a string.
I twist and turn at my parents' whim.

And at each teacher's request,
I genuflect and reply.

My coach says run!
I ask how fast? How far?

The choirmaster shouts:
"Sing! Sing as if your life depended on it."
I do. It does.

I deny myself in order to be free.

5'4" and 90 pounds

Is that your only concern?

Voice Over

"Mrs. Thomas, I'm so sorry."

&

She begins calm and collected, recounting her son's achievements with a reporter's accuracy. She concludes collapsing under the weight of the awful.

&&

This is the first of three poems portraying a mother's attempt to reconcile the presence of evil in a world created by a beneficent God. Job struggled and a satisfactory answer has yet to appear.

Dreams

He was going to college - first in the family. We were so proud of him.

He was going to be a doctor - like you, taking care of any and all.

He read all the time and wrote.
Shakespeare, Wordsworth, Poe - You would think they were his classmates,
the way he talked about them.

And what an athlete! No one could outrun or outjump him.
In this here county, no one ever ran the mile faster.

He flew 20 feet off the cliff, before he began to fall.
Doctor at UT says when you break your neck, there is no pain.

I disagree. I cry every day.

Voice Over

"Ben, How can I be of assistance today?"

&

Ben's anger cannot be ignored or minimized. He wants answers to unanswerable questions, and his frequent references to directions only underscore how lost and confused he is.

&&

In this first of two poems, this young man, like Debra (Mission Trip), is forced to rewrite his life and plan new goals. Some people when dealt a hard blow, collapse in defeat; others will rise to new heights of achievement. And it is very difficult to predict an individual's response.

Wrong Turn

If I had turned right instead of left,
Life would be alright.
But having turned left,
My world, in an instant, exploded and I am left to pick up all the pieces.

I was a carpenter - now what am I?
How many one-armed carpenters does it take to frame a house?
No one knows - it has never been done!
What is the difference between a one-armed man and an empty beer can?
The latter can at least be recycled!

My fiancee left me.
She says she needs to hug a whole man.
And my screams at night awaken her.
She once loved me dearly but now I am different.
And she cannot love a stranger.

She does me wrong.
Is that right?

Voice Over

"Mr. Jeffers, Today, how goes life?"

He is still reeling in pain afraid that it will never end. His voice conveys a fear that is palpable. But even in the darkest of storms the soft whistle of a bird called Hope can be heard. The poem ends on such a note.

To Heal

It takes but a moment to shred another's soul,
Toss its pieces to the winds and shrug indifferently.
Frantic with fear,
Faint with pain,
I search knowing full well there are fragments never ever to be found.
It takes much, much more than time to mend a broken heart:
Wisdom to understand.
Courage to forgive. Patience to heal.

Voice Over

"Mrs. Bell, How can I help?"

This is a complicated woman and not very likeable. It is clear that she has been a frequent visitor to the office, demanding much, appreciative never.

Her symptoms elude diagnosis until the second to the last line. At that moment, the reader senses just how intense her pain truly is. But she does not yet have the courage to express it. And her hasty retort makes it nigh impossible to extend a hand.

Hypochondriasis is the focus of many jokes. We laugh heartedly in order to avoid thoughtful consideration of the condition's causes. To do so would be too threatening to our emotional equilibrium. The financial consequences of untreated or mistreated psychosomatic illness is staggering.

Answers

Good news? All tests normal?
CBC, CCP, UA, MRI, EMG, NCV, CT.
You know more about me than any man has right to learn.

So why do I walk like a rag doll on a stick - lurching and reeling; As if I stand
upon a ship at sea, with waves crashing against its bow?

In my head - of course - but not the way you so imply.

Do you think I like my plight?
Unable to work, incapable of caring for my kids, can't even make love.
All I can do is sit and let others minister to me (not that I don't deserve it).

If I had money, I'd find a real doc!

Voice Over

"Jennifer, please sit down."

This unfortunate young lady is literally gasping in anguish as she tries to contemplate a future she never ever imagined. The destructiveness of her actions overwhelms her, yet trying to reverse course would be even more criminal. She sits helpless without a sense of hope.

The prefrontal cortex, the center of rational thought, is not fully developed until the person reaches their early 20's. Thus behavior that to an adult is illogical can control the actions of youth. Abstinence only programs don't work because they are predicated on logical behavior.

Mistakes

No way!
No way!

It cannot be. He said - "in and out quickly"
And it will not be.

My life is ruined.
My father's also.
He'll kill me if I don't flee.

What should I do?
What should I do?

I'll abort. No. What crime did my child commit to deserve execution?
I'll run, bear the baby, then walk away.

I didn't even like the boy.
We did it on a dare.

How can I create a life?
When I have yet to live one?

Voice Over

"Mr. Dunn, Let me talk to you."

In seconds, he envisions the grand sweep of his life and with a quiet and dignified demeanor, surveys the difficult territory he must now traverse.

Unlike Mr. Bolt (Cut and Deal), Mr. Dunn confronts the inevitable with remarkable calmness. Is it because he is deeply religious and believes that God moves us from one stage to another at his choosing or are there other sources of his courage? This is the first of three poems to explore his psyche.

Six Letters - Part 1

Hello Doc!
What say the tests?
Lay it straight

Cancer?

Funny how that little word stills the beating heart and chills the
marrow to its deepest core.
I know I have a fighting chance,
Yet, I feel I have lost it all.

Now, the distant horizons of my future,
Seem but an arm's length from my grasp.
And years of revelry and rest, pleasurable pursuits,
Will be replaced by frantic months of tying knots.

Funny how life turns on six letters.

Voice Over

"Mr. Johnson, And what brings you to my door today?"

There are men with such a jovial nature that all who cross their path cannot help but smile - all day. He does not deny reality. He accepts it all and loves every portion of it.

There are men with such a jovial nature that all who cross their path cannot help but smile - all day. He does not deny reality. He accepts it all and loves every portion of it.

A Jewish psychiatrist, Victor Frankel, survivor of a concentration camp in WWII, remarked that everything can be taken from a man but one possession - the attitude with which he chooses to confront his fate.

Wingdinger

I need my wingdinger checked.
That's what the cardiologist said - every month.
Actually, he called it a pacemaker but given what it does for me,
It certainly needs a name with more pizzazz.

Doc, I have eight conditions not counting old age and loneliness.
Today, I'm in a generous mood -you can have two; no questions asked.

You hear about the old woman arrested for shoplifting a can of peaches?
Judge asked her why.
"I was hungry" was her reply.
"The law requires I sentence you a day in jail for each of six slices."

The husband now rose.
"Honor, may I have a word?"

"Yes you may. What will you say?"
"She also stole a can of peas."

Doc, if you don't keep laughing, you'll drown in your own tears.

Voice Over

"Mr. Lessing, How goes things?"

A melancholy recollection laced with wistfulness characterizes this gentleman's initial comments. Then anger erupts as he recounts the cruel strokes of misfortune that struck down his wife. And it ends with a question and a promise that informs the doctor of the path Mr. Lessing is contemplating.

An American Indian proverb states it so succinctly:
Do not judge a man until you have walked in his moccasins. So let us suspend our opinion for awhile and watch.

Morpheus

Good afternoon, Doc.
How is Grace? Not well and this is why I have come.

You didn't know her in her youth but she was quite a looker.
Many have asked me how I - plain-faced and short - could have
captured such a prize.
I told them with a wink and nod, that it's not how you look
but what you do that matters.
And oh, the back-slaps I would get.

She seemed to all so demurely shy and sweet,
But let me tell you -
I can recall as if yesterday how she sat upon me and rode me as a cowgirl.
And I screamed,
And I shouted,
And I laughed,
And I cried as she bent me to her will.
I loved her more than anything else - even more than my health.
Long walks holding her hand.
Smelling her hair as I brushed my nose across her nape.
There is heaven on earth, don't let anyone tell you otherwise.

Then came the cancer.
I didn't miss the breast but she did, and once a thought plants itself in a
woman's head, not even dynamite can dislodge it.
So shamed by her disfigurement, she hid from me; and at my touch, recoiled.

Then the stroke and half a body went, and all her mind.
Now once a beauty to behold, lay shriveled, pale and mute.

There are times she seems in so much pain.

Doc, did you know that morphine comes from Morpheus, the
Greek god of sleep?
You do?
Ah, then let us talk some more.

Voice Over

"Dan, you seem quite agitated. What is the problem?"

This man acts aggrieved, as if his integrity is being impugned. He simply cannot see or perhaps refuses to acknowledge another way of interpreting his behavior. There is also a hint that he has a right to behave this way. And just who are you to question?

The capacity of a human being to act in a way, that in their heart of hearts, they recognize as fundamentally wrong is boundless. The psychiatrists call it rationalization. But as the farmers say, "The chickens will come home to roost."

An Affair-1

My wife thinks I am having an affair,
But I'm not!

Yet, like the question - have you stopped beating your wife?
Any answer implicates and indicts.

Yes, I have a friend - a special friend.
It is true that I blush at every compliment, And laugh at all her jokes,
And yes, I catch my breath at inadvertent touch.
But we have not had sex - so no affair!

We share much: our problems, our hopes, our fears and aspirations.
But we have not had sex - so no affair!

Yes we tease and insinuate but these are harmless jokes that refresh the day.
Yes we communicate frequently and rendezvous at conferences
Unbeknownst to our respective spouses.
But we have not had sex - so no affair!

Why would I have an affair?
And destroy all that I love and live for?
That makes no sense.
And sense is what I have an abundance of.

Voice Over

"William, Good day my friend."

As he straightens up the room's furnishings, one cannot help but smile. He does seem a little odd, but in no way bothered by his idiosyncrasies.

Obsessive compulsive disorder is "characterized by uncontrollable obsessions and compulsions, which the sufferer usually recognizes as being excessive or unreasonable." This definition does not even remotely reflect the turbulent storms that rage through a patient's psyche. This, the first of four poems, is light. No others will be.

First Things First

Hello Doc,
I'm doing fine.

Excuse the interruption but
Your papers are askew,
As is the diploma and carpet too.

What is the matter sir?

You know my thoughts run ragged, if lines are so.

Voice Over
"Mrs. Strong, Please, we have a lot to discuss."

Outrage, pure and simple outrage, assails the physician's ears. She speaks for all those parents who learn that their child has a terrible affliction. First, they question the establishment's authority to label and therefore control. Then they describe their child's condition from a totally different perspective. So who is right?

How a society defines behavior and categorizes pathology is not simply the province of science. Consider homosexuality and reflect upon the actions of politicians and religious leaders who refuse to stand quietly on the sidelines. It is my belief that the less we know about the origins of a condition, which some are inclined to call deviant, the more involved non-scientists become.

Autism

So, you say my son is autistic?

Upon his brow, you have now stamped the letter A, as if this mark
reflected heinous crime.
And what foul deed did he commit to so deserve this tragic fate?

My son inhabits a universe to which we have no key,
A world beyond our understanding,
A planet beyond our reach.
He sees things you would never dare to face and nor would I.
With this soft brush, I gently stroke his nape, and he cries as if
A thousand blades had raked his skin.
I whisper and the cannons boom.
And the fragrance of a single petal carries him to Heaven's gates.
He speaks in tongue and I to him.
Now who is poet and who is scribe?

Who gives you the right to name and sort?
Are you Linnaeus?
My son stands outside your ordered universe
And to your authority, will neither bend his knee nor bow his head.

Voice Over

"Mr. Bolt, How can I help you today?"

&

He begins calmly as a good negotiator should. Then becomes plaintive when the first approach fails, And finally erupts in anger hoping that intimidation will turn the tide.

&&

It is very painful from a physician's point of view, to watch a man struggle against the knowledge of imminent defeat. There really is nothing he can offer but a willingness to stand by his side. In the future, he will be useful.

Cut And Deal - Part 2

I'm back, so let us renegotiate.
I need to buy some time - too much to do
50 grand for one year?
100 K for two?

Is there not in your black bag,
A potion that can stretch time?
Is there not, upon your desk, a magic pen that can rewrite fate?

Just give me the goddamn bill!
Just give me the goddamn bill!

Voice Over

"Mrs. Filston, You seem pretty upset. What is bothering you?"

❧

She is really angry and frustrated at her mind's weakness. How could it treat her so disrespectfully? And you, doctor, better repair it!

❧❧

What frightens us more - the loss of body functions or the stumbling of our minds? From my experience, people fear the latter far more than the former. I think it reflects the belief that our minds, not our bodies, define us.

Memory

Doc,
It's my memory!
Events from distant years are as sharp as yesterday's news.
While events just past, seem obscured by mists of time.

I make lists - I lose the lists.
Twice a week, at least, I lose my keys
And turn the house inside out until I ultimately find them - always in the last
place I look.

A specific example? Here's one.

Several weeks ago, while working in the garden,
I placed my cellphone, not having pockets, in my waistband.
I soon got busy and unnoticed, the phone slipped into my pants.
Hours passed and when I finished, it was nowhere to be found.
Frantic and furious, I searched and in frustration sought my husband's aid.

"Honey, how difficult must you make this problem?
Just stand in the yard, and listen for my call."

Doc,
Don't you dare go there!
And for the record, it was not on vibrate.

Voice Over

"Mrs. Thomas, Is there anything I can do?"

What can one say in the face of such overwhelming grief? Her grief becomes yours and there are no words of comfort.

Gone

How can one ever hope to understand the inconceivable or
comprehend the senseless?
In despair, I raise my voice and implore the Heavens for an answer.

But only silence, a deafening silence, greets my ears.

Grief gnaws at my heart
And anguish camps at my doorstep.

Voice Over

"Mr. Wilson, An unexpected problem delayed me. I am sorry I'm late."

He is so obnoxious and so damn condescending! The only way you can tolerate him is to believe that you, like Job, are being tested.

Busy Man - Part 2

Doc,

You're 15 minutes late and my blood pressure is still too high.

I have fired VP's for less.
Look,
I'm in a generous mood today.
We'll cut a deal.

Your bill is on the house and I won't charge you for my wasted time.

Voice Over

"William, I cannot help but notice a look of discomfort."

&

His desperation is palpable and his fear of self destruction is beginning to emerge.

.

&&

When the mind turns upon itself, there is no place to hide.

A Spider's Web (OCD)

My thoughts ensnare me as a spider's web a fly,
And as I struggle to disentangle, tighter grow the bonds.

I would, if I could, will these thoughts away,
But the very act of mind drives imprint even deeper.

"Out, out damn spot"
Lady M and I could share a beer and curse our common fate.

But unlike her, I am imprisoned by my mind for a crime I have no
knowledge of.

Voice Over
"Mrs. Rolston, Are things any better these days?"

She has no insight and doubtful ever will. Just one long whining complaint or demand after another. Listening to a nail scrape across a blackboard is music to one's ears compared to the bleating of this woman.

There are patients, and every physician will admit this, who are thoroughly unlikeable. Before you walk into the room, you need to ready yourself by reciting the Oath of Hippocrates. To help someone like this, one must suppress all emotion.

Tough Times

Doc, I just don't feel well.
And I think the Prozac is messin' with my head.

I'm tired all the time - irritated and agitated.
The slightest provocation sets me off.
Restful sleep is a dream never fulfilled.
I taste nothing and nothing gives me pleasure.
Sex? What is that?

How's my husband? He has yet to get a job, that lazy SOB.
He says he has no allergies but whenever he finds work
He breaks out in a rash and gets sick.
If he worked ½ the time he spent whining about his back, we would be rich.

My son? Out of jail next year.
5 years is far too hard a punishment for breaking and entering an empty house.
No one got hurt and he only took what the owners didn't need. Anyway, that lady
got all her jewelry back, and the insurance company paid for repairs.

My daughter? Has given me 5 beautiful grandchildren.
Unfortunately they come attached to three losers - if she's smart, she'll divorce the
third just like the other two.

Don't hassle me about my weight.
I have carried 100 extra pounds for 20 years so I'm used to it.
And I watch what I put in my mouth - a bird would not
survive on what I eat.

Yes, I smoke 2 packs a day.
It is nothing about which I am ashamed.
My old man says all the hype about tobacco is nothing more than a liberal
conspiracy designed to destroy American jobs and take away the rights of God-
fearing people.

Doc, I need a nighttime potty - so I don't have to walk to the bathroom. I'm getting
up a lot to pee and that makes me mighty tired.
Also need a sticker for my car- so I can park right
by the entrance of the store.
I exercise daily- walk the length of my driveway to pick up mail - so I'm doing all the
right things.

You can't imagine how I suffer so. The Prozac is just not working.
Give me something that does and make sure it's covered –
I ain't paying a cent for my medicine if I don't have to.

Voice Over

"Mr. May, I have not seen you for awhile."

❧

Exasperation and an aggrieved sense of entitlement is how he announces his decision. He remembers what he once had, acknowledges honestly what he now has but nonetheless finds insufficient.

❧❧

All marriages, even between the most compatible of pairs, enter periods of real trial and doubt. Many crumble under the weight of this crisis. To avoid this, they must do three things:

Accept that the past cannot be recaptured, for a new relationship is unique. Believe that the future can be better, for a long term relationship is also unique. Never forget the present, for problems ignored do not disappear.

Moving On

I have had enough.
Time to go,
Twenty years of unhappiness.

Not really.
When we met, I thought she "hung the moon."
Each time we touched, my heart raced.
Butterflies took up residence in my chest
And my loins ached for hers.

She is truly a good woman, thoughtful, kind and sweet.
Attentive to each and all of my wishes. She cares deeply for me.
And I for her.

But what was fire in my heart now simply smolders.
Though embers flicker now and then, there is little heat
And less light.

So we part.
One chapter in my life now closes, its last sheet
Stained with tears.
A new one begins - blank pages yet to be written.

Voice Over
> *"Mrs. May, I understand that all is not well in your life."*

&

Resignation, a sense of defeat, and a determination not to lose again.

&&

If she and her husband had only been honest and unburdened their souls, how different it would have been.

Freedom - Part 1

I have had enough.
Time to go,
Twenty years of unhappiness.

Not really.
When we met, I thought he "hung the moon."
Each time we touched, my heart raced.
Butterflies took up residence in my chest
And my loins ached for his.

He is truly a good man, thoughtful, kind and sweet.
Attentive to each and all of my wishes. He cares deeply for me.
And I for him.

But what was fire in my heart now simply smolders.
Though embers flicker now and then, there is little heat.
And less light.

So we part.
One chapter in my life now closes, its last sheet
Stained with tears.
A new one begins - blank pages yet to be written.

Voice Over

"Dan, you look terrible. Sit down."

The "chickens have come home to roost."

This man who once was supremely confident, almost arrogantly so, is now a trembling child, seeking answers.

Some lessons should be learned only by listening. Learning by experience is just too painful.

An Affair - Part 2

My wife has caught me in a lie,
And my world implodes upon itself.

I will never forget her look
As anguish etched itself across her face.
Like a fault-line slowly separating earth at its edges,
all tumbling into the abyss.

My marriage is like a train in freefall off a bridge
And when it strikes the ground,
Its passengers - those that live - will be forever maimed.

Love, sex, commitment - I thought they had nothing to do with one another.
But no! They have everything to do with each other.

Voice Over
> *"Mr. Tate, Your wife warned me of your coming. I'm sure you have a different take."*

His joy of life cannot be denied. The energy exudes from every pore of his body. Even as he recounts his disasters, he cannot help but laugh.

Like Mr. Johnson (Wingdinger), there are people who appear to be congenitally programmed to wring out of every experience a dram of pleasure. Biologists have yet to discover that gene. The elixir of youth lies within and not in the Florida swamps.

Accidents

Hello Doc.
I'm here for an ER follow up - third time in three months.
My wife says I'm an "accident waiting to happen";
Not true. I'm just unlucky.

When you clean a room, you need to vacuum the curtains.
Not my fault the rods couldn't hold me.

I love to boat - have done so for thirty years.
How was I to know my friend forgot to tie the bow when
I stepped off the dock?

Do you realize that not all the sidewalks in Atlantic City
have ramps for wheelchairs?
So I missed a step and slipped.
Is that a crime?

My wife says that I am 70 and should stop acting as if
the decimal point was to the left of the zero.
You're as young or as old as you choose to be.
The body follows a willing spirit.

Now, do not tell my wife that this question I asked –
What happens to a pacemaker when one bungee jumps?

Voice Over

"Miss Beulah, is it not a beautiful day?"

Like a train without brakes barreling down a mountain, Miss Beulah levels all who have the misfortune of crossing the tracks as she passes by. Passengers can only hold tight and pray she does not crash.

The physician has two options when he confronts such a patient. He can fight back and try to control the conversation - a losing proposition, or he can sit back and listen and simply try to enjoy the experience.

Why am I Here?

Doc, why am I here?
You don't have the time to listen.

In July, I got a bill from Medicare for work done 6 months before.
(They move slower than molasses in January - that I know for sure.)
But it was more than I really owed according to my friend, Gladys.

Did you realize that Gladys got breast cancer one month ago?
Never wanted to get a mammogram but I insisted.
Praise the Lord for my persistence.

Anyway I called Medicare 23 times last month and never
did get a straight answer.
So I am not paying it. They can put me behind bars as far as I care.
Are you still the jail doc? Then you can see me there.
I hear there is no smoking - can I have a patch?

I realize I lost weight. Now don't go rushing me.
Alice says (who's Alice? - she's my hairdresser)
That the reason is I'm worrying about my brother Bob who has been laid off.
He used to work for the county
but when the new manager was hired, "he cleaned house."
I think it was 'cause Bob's a Democrat and I hear the manager ain't.
I think it is a cryin' shame that politics gets in the way of good government.
Don't you?
Isn't Senator Anna Belle your mother-in-law?
Maybe she can pull some strings.

How much do I eat? 3 meals a day. But only 2 on Monday, Wednesday and
Friday cause that's when the TV show {do you watch TV?) Lost Love comes
on and I get so choked up that I can't digest my meal so I skip it.

So what can you do for me today?
Well if you stop interrupting and pay attention I'll tell you.
So Gladys came over a couple of days ago to show me her mastectomy scar -
and it's a "beaut".
If I have to have a mastectomy, you need to send me to Dr. Morgan.
Anyway, she was showin' me the exercises she needs to do - "walkin' her
hand up the wall" (like this) and I was wearing a blouse I got from the

Sweetwater Flea Market. They have a lot of good stuff. And you don't have to pay what the seller asks. You can always "Jew him down".

The blouse was a size too large (I had lost 10 lbs, just like you told me to at the last visit). So when I reached up, the blouse came off my back.
And Gladys cried
"God sakes alive, you have a mole the size of a buffalo nickel on your back."
And I says How should I know?
Do I have eyes on the back of my head?

I just got a pair of fancy readin' glasses from the new optometrist but they only work for the eyes next to my nose. (By the way, he has a real nice office - good music, glossy magazines, and even serves coffee. His wife is the receptionist, but "bless her heart", she is as ugly as a toad).

So if you have time, could you take it off? Or I could come back tomorrow.

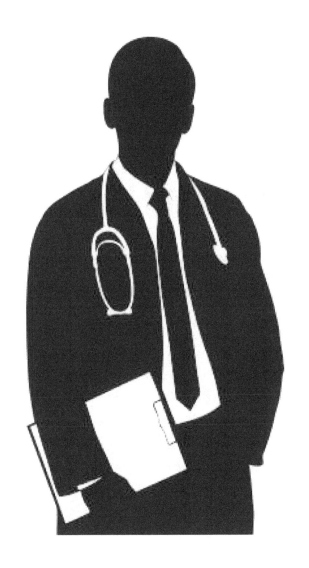

Voice Over

"Lonnie, so what is on your agenda?"

&

Matter-of-fact, no emotion until the end.

&&

To cross paths with a psychopath unnerves even the most experienced of practitioners. The amoral self-centeredness leaves one gasping for fresh air. We don't hesitate to kill a rabid dog. Are there not rabid people also?

The Thumb

It's my thumb, Doc.
I think I strained it strangling that asshole who couldn't keep his mouth shut.

He accused me of fuckin' his wife.
You ever see his old lady? She's so fat you need a pole
and a miner's lamp to plumb her.
I should've walked.

But then, he said that the only way I could get it up was to tie a
rope to an over-head pulley and yank.
No one makes fun of my manhood and lives to talk about it.

It isn't easy to choke a man to death,
'specially if he has a size 24" neck and he's not cooperating.
You can tell when the light is about to go out.
The gleam in his eyes fades,
The pupils narrow to a pin and then explode.

God, I never felt so full of life as when I took another's.

But let's get back to my thumb, Doc.

Voice Over

"Mr. Jeffers, your face tells a story and it seems so sad."

&

He is so sad. For though a person can be forgiven, their actions cannot be forgotten. Innocence once lost can never be recovered.

&&

A broken heart heals no more quickly than a shattered leg. There are many pieces that need to be melded together. The orthopedist inserts screws to hasten his work's completion. Were there such for the heart?

Reverie

We have spent our passion and now in the quiet stillness of night, lay upon
sheets wet, warm, and crumpled.
Cooled by the whirling draft of the overhead,
You slumber peacefully exhausted.
Sleep has folded her arms about you and the gentle rhythm of your breath
lulls me.

Minutes before, your gasps and cries filled my ears and I succumbed
willingly, gratefully
to the urgent thrusts of your thighs.
Your arms clasped me and I was yours.

But I cannot forget your letter to a friend -
Promising teasingly, playfully, a weekend of wine, bed and body –
Pleasures beyond measure,
Delights beyond number.
And the residue of distrust, turns bitter the honey of your lips.

My dreams lay shattered at my feet - innocence lost
Sleep turns her back, indifferent to my weary soul.

Voice Over

"Mr. Langley, how can I help today?"

This man is truly confused and asks for help in a straightforward manner. As a late aside, he makes one more request and therein lay the answer.

&·&·

One of my residency professors, an old family physician by the name of Bill Wilson, said that medicine is very easy. If you listen to your patient carefully, he will eventually reveal the source of his misery. The trick is to settle back and hear him out.

Headache

Doc,
I have a headache whose nature I do not understand.
It appears without provocation - day or night.

No aura announces its arrival; no other symptom stands at its side.
It can be here, there or everywhere.

Sometimes it lasts mere seconds; at other times it will linger for hours –
not severe, but always on my mind.
Nothing makes it worse and nothing makes it better.
It just departs on its own accord.

Exam is normal? I knew this is what you'd say.
Perhaps, I'll return another day.

One last request.
I know your time is short and many clamor for your ear.
I need a sleeping pill.
Last month I learned my wife has cancer and there is no cure.

Voice Over
"Cynthia, I am in no rush. What is the matter?"

&

Grief and fear grip her soul. She begs for respite. Time is running out.

&&

Depression is a killer. Suicide ranks as one of the leading causes of death among adolescents. To witness an internal assault upon the human psyche is no less frightful than watching an avalanche shred a mountainside. And a physician cannot help but feel that turning back the rock slide might be easier than saving his patient.

Voices

The voices!
They harass, humiliate, harangue, and haunt me.
"You are a failure."
"You never were or will be worthwhile."

They jeer and sneer.
"You misbegotten soul. Conceived in error, Born by accident.
You take up space and waste air."

They condescend and condemn.
"Kill yourself! Feed a worm
And achieve in death what in life you never will - a purpose."

My mind has turned upon itself
Runs riot through the brain.
And Hope, defenseless, drowns in a pool of misery.

Voice Over

"Ben, you look different today."

He speaks in a defiant and victorious voice - He is down but not out.

&&

Nietzsche said "That which does not kill us only makes us stronger."
Ben may not have read the philosopher but nonetheless personifies his
opinion. If there is a gene for optimism, could there not also be one for grit.

Frog

So she thinks I'm less a man for being short an arm?
Then what is she, who lacks a heart?

Yes, I have been cut down.
My knees and forehead burrowed in the mud.
And breath comes hard and slow.
But still-I live!

I'm like the frog who by chance misfortune,
Slips into a vat of milk.
The sides are smooth, too slick to climb;
So all he can do is paddle.

Hours pass and slowly to the bottom drifts frog,
Mindful of his fate.
Then a voice rings out - Not now, not yet!
And to the surface, once more he swims.

The night is very long - the hours longer.
But when the morning sun rises to front
The crimson dawn,
Upon a pad of butter, sits the frog to introduce the pair.

Rivit Rivit Rivit

Voice Over

"Mr. Jeffers, life is still difficult. Your face tells me so."

&

He is so tired of the struggle. He wants desperately resolution but he is not sure that with time it will come.

&&

What is the different between needing a person and wanting a person? Can you need a person and not want them? Can you want a person whom you do not need? And how does one know when a person you need wants you?

Memories

Six months have passed and time has yet to heal the wound.
But simply lays a film across the ugly tear obscuring from casual witness
deeper truth.

A day does not pass when thoughts of my humiliation do not throttle my
soul and anger wells up in my breast
Like heat from a volcano smoldering silently beneath a thin crust of dirt.

I hate myself for hating her.
I hate myself for hating him.
I hate myself.

I know she needs me.
What I need to know is whether she wants me.

Voice Over

"Mr. Dunn, you look full of spirit today."

&

Exuberance, confidence, macho, bravado. He will prevail, no doubt about that.

&&

There is much to admire in a man who refuses to throw in the towel. One cannot help but feel embarrassed by one's own weaknesses and insecurities. Patients seldom realize how much an impact they have upon physicians. And physicians are reluctant to admit so. Why? I wish I knew.

Six Letters - Part 2

Hello Doc!
Like my new "do"?

Dr. Volpe, the cancer doc, (she's quite a looker)
Says I'm "devastatingly handsome"
(Yup, those are her exact words.)

Says also that if anyone can lick this disease,
It's me.
Why?

Cause I'm a fighter and
I'm from Tennessee
And I can't spell surrender.

Voice Over

"Mrs. Finch, let me hear you out for there are questions I will need to ask".

She is a pragmatist first and foremost. She gives a non-nonsense accounting of what she must do in order to survive.

Domestic violence statistics don't tell half the story, but they do reflect a plague no less destructive than the Bubonic.

One-third of American women are assaulted by their partner during their lifetime. Millions of women receive serious and sometimes life threatening injuries annually from their male partner.

Most women who die do so at the hands of someone they know.

'Til Death Do Us Part

Seventeen years - I love him.
You don't understand because you don't know.

My father was a nasty man - beat my mother everyday
And would one day have killed her,
Had not a car spared him the effort.

I raised my two younger sisters. Father was too busy drinkin' and chasin'
women to care for the three he had at home.

When I turned sixteen, Richard appeared.
Promised me "a castle in the clouds."
Wouldn't you go if you had been living all
Your life in a dungeon?

He cares about me.
Calls me every hour to make sure I'm OK.
Makes sure he knows who my friends are - lots of "bad influences" out there.
Gives me money to buy what I need but not more.

Sex? Every day.
Sometimes I'm too tired.
Sometimes I hafta do things I wish I didn't.
(I'll spare you the details, Doc.)
But this is a small price to pay for a roof over one's
head and food on the table.

Does he drink?
Yes, but he's a man and can hold it - most of the time.

Seventeen years - I love him.
I just wish he'd take off the ring before he hits me.

Voice Over

"Hello, Mrs. Arnett, what brings us to together today?"

&

She voices her thoughts with an air of wonderment. She is not sure from where the wellsprings of her love arise nor could she ever have imagined herself acting as she now does.

&&

One of the great mysteries of life - the origin of unconditional love.

The Workings of the Heart

When we first met, he could shoulder the world with a casual shrug.
He knew no fear, for in his words, "There was nothing to fear."
We cycled the countryside, daring the curves with reckless abandon.

And the sex!
To be held so tight that I could hardly breathe.
To be so completely overwhelmed.
I cried and laughed and shouted and screamed.
I lived to die in his arms.

Now I organize his pills - 18 at last count - in neat little boxes.
Checking at the end of the day, for their absence - For he is a tad forgetful.

He gets lost easily, so we always park on the same side of the store.
When he falls out of bed, I gently raise him up.

This is not what I envisioned nor what I bargained for.
Yet, my love for him grows ever deeper.

The workings of the heart are so strange.
Are they not?

Voice Over

"Debra, So nice to see you again."

She is a changed woman. When first we met, she was a naive waif crushed by the gratuitous cruelty of amoral men. Now she appears strong and confident, secure in the knowledge that she was tested by God and not found wanting.

Tragedy befalls us all. Why does one person succumb and another use it to catapult herself to a higher plane of existence? I doubt we will ever fully understand the determinants of our character.

Mystery

Yes, I plan to return. Why not?

I have felt the icy grip of terror clasp my throat.
Now I can peer into another's eyes, see nameless fear
And steady their soul.

I have shouldered crushing grief.
Now I can hear another's cry of pain And offer balm.

Anguish once blotted out all thought.
Now I can grasp the hand of a lost and
Frightened man and hold tight

That is why.

Oh, my child. I'll name her Mystery —
For who among us can God's ways divine?

Voice Over
"Dr. Barnes, this is a surprise. What can I do for you today?"

&

The doctor is overwhelmed by feelings of sadness. He finally recognizes his perilous state and knows that without help, his future is dim. He is so scared that pride no longer inhibits him.

&&

Physicians have a very difficult time admitting either fault or failure. They live in a society that wants to believe that they are infallible. This adulation is like a coat of armor - at times protective of our psyches but at other times, so heavy that it weighs us down, precluding rational thought and prudent action.

Doctor

It's hard for a doc to see a doc,
To hear advice that he himself dispenses daily.

But there is more to my reluctance than simply that.

I am weary in a way for which there is no measure.
I struggle daily simply to care.

You'd never guess by my façade,
My face - a mask that hides the truth.

But the effort to sustain the lie now exceeds my will.

And that is why I'm here today.

Voice Over

"Mr. Crisp, you don't look very good today."

He talks as if the very act of speaking requires more energy than humanly possible. Bewildered, frustrated, exhausted - he cannot imagine an end to his misery.

For those romantics who find depression an alluring state of being, I advise a conversation with someone so afflicted. Their face is a portrait of sorrow, their voice a dirge, their words one long cry of helplessness and hopelessness. One feels their own energy being sucked into an emotional black hole.

The Walls of Jericho

The heavy hands of fatigue rest upon my shoulders
And lean and lean and lean
Until beneath their weight my knees begin to buckle.

Speech is labor and rational thought a hopeless task.

I mark the hours of the day upon my rising
And bribe the clock to speed its passage on its daily circuit.

I hug my pillow as if I were a drowning man thrown a piece of flotsam.
Then my mind awakens - and everything I did that day,
Or failed to do or must do on the morrow,
Marches relentlessly through my brain,
Like Joshua's army 'round the walls of Jericho,
Trumpeting its message until I, like them, collapse.

Is there not a pill to erase the ledger and turn off the circuits?
Is there not a drug which, at the break of day, can start my engine?
Is there not a nostrum to make me want
to dance, to sing, to laugh and to love?

"William, has the medicine helped?"

This young man is becoming increasingly desperate. He knows that once the salmon is brought to the deck, life slips away quickly.

Obsessive-Compulsive disorder is terrifying in its relentless assault upon the patient's sanity. It is truly a war within and because one can hide no secrets from himself, the advantage rests with the foe.

On Fish and Thoughts

My mind plays me as a fisherman grappling with a salmon.

I struggle to disengage the barbs that pin me tightly to the line.

But with each twist and turn, they burrow deeper;

For my mind, like a fisherman, knows
All the tricks.

Voice Over

"Mr. Jeffers, you look better today. Is it true or simply show?"

&

Hope wages war with doubt. And the contest within one's mind hangs in the balance.

&&

When trust is lost, all actions can be subjected to the most cynical of interpretations. The constant to and fro - Does she love me or does she not - amusing when a 7-year-old plucks a daisy, is an exhausting exercise for an adult. And the question - Will it ever end? - hovers continuously in the recesses of the mind, sapping even more energy.

The Play - Act 1

You act as if you
Admire
Respect
Honor
Love
Cherish
And desire me.
Thus I am reassured until I wonder if it is
Just an act.

Voice Over

"Mrs. May, what is on your mind today?"

The poem begins as a paean to independence. She is in total command and revels in her new found strength. But doubt begins to infiltrate her mind as she describes her ex- husband's behavior. It ends with the tragic admission that the price of freedom can be steep.

It is a continual struggle in even the most harmonious of marriages - how to accommodate each partner's need for independence (which includes the right to choose their own friends) and the other partner's reasonable expectations that there are boundaries on acceptable behavior. What one can do as a spouse is more circumscribed than the actions of a single person.

Freedom - Part 2

I'm free!
Free at last!
I am a woman - hear my song.
I ask nothing of anyone,
And none asks anything of me.

Sex?
I take when I need it,
And when finished, walk.

Friends?
I have many - too many to count.
Friends to dine with.
Friends to ski with.
Friends to sing with.

My ex?
He's moved on and found another.
(How dare he so soon!)
She's not perfect (I'm certainly prettier).
But he says,
"I never sought perfection for blemish mars us all."
He's content, I see it in his eyes.

Doc,
I'm alone and so lonely.

Voice Over

"Mr. Armstrong, you are full of spirit today!"

The joyful mood of a convert reverberates off the walls. Having seen the Promised Land, there is no turning back. And the more people he can convince to come, the better.

The joyful mood of a convert reverberates off the walls. Having seen the Promised Land, there is no turning back. And the more people he can convince to come, the better.

Unfortunately, many people view science and religion as adversarial systems of thought. It is a pathetic farce when Creationists debate the merits of Darwin's Theory of Evolution. It is tragic beyond measure, when the advancements of medicine - drugs surgery, radiation therapy - are refused on the grounds that reliance upon them implies a rejection of God. Each year, countless die because prayer alone did not cure.

Saved

You'll be proud to hear I gave up smokin', drinkin' and fornicatin'.
Turned over a new leaf, yes sir, new chapter bein' written.

Found Jesus three Sundays ago, and life is sure sweet.
I know you don't believe in Him. That's a shame,
'cause I hate to see a good man go to Hell.

Came by to say I no longer need to see you.
Goin' to save a heap of money - no need to buy medicines or pay for tests.

The Good Book says: "Trust in the Lord and upon the
wings of angels shall ye soar."

AMEN.

Voice Over

"Janet, I have difficult news to share."

This young lady is struggling with the unavoidable fact that her behavior was incomprehensibly stupid and henceforth, she will have to suffer the consequences. For some actions, there are no "do-overs".

This young lady is struggling with the unavoidable fact that her behavior was incomprehensibly stupid and henceforth, she will have to suffer the consequences. For some actions, there are no "do-overs".

When discussing risky behavior (drugs, alcohol, sex) with teenagers, I am astonished by their nearly universal belief that bad things will not happen to them. It is their delusion of invincibility that is so hard to break; if we could, there would be far fewer tears.

And I'll Die Soon

So this is how it ends.
It would be funny, were the joke not on me.

He didn't seem the type.
I know there isn't such a thing as type.
But nonetheless, he didn't seem the type.

White, so handsome and so very educated.
He wined and dined me- swept me off my feet.
Prince Charming would have wept in shame.

He left no address - no way, therefore, to track him down.
I'm sure he knows - how could he not?

So this is how it ends.
A broken condom in the hands of Death.
The stuff of life, my poison potion.

And I'll Die Soon.

"Mr. Bolt, how can I be of assistance?"

Calm resignation is the tone he conveys until the end when once again, he demands the means to assert himself - true to character.

As I discuss with my patients Advance Directives/Living Wills, I am struck by the similarity of requests. People ask not for the application of every piece of technology at medicine's disposal. Rather, it is the wish that one die as a solitary human being and not as an appendage to a machine.

Cut and Deal - Part 3

It appears to my chagrin, that this is one fight I'm not destined to win.
Few have ever bested me, yet now, I understand
I will not raise my hand in victory.

It was a good fight though little did I realize how
much advantage rested with my foe.

I am not complaining nor should any weep.
But when I exit, let me choose the time and place.

And so, I come today with one request.
Do not let me die in pain whimpering for anodyne.
Give me means to end my life quick - and with dignity and grace.

Voice Over

"Mr. Dunn, you look very tired today."

With a rueful smile and a casual shrug that belies the solemnity of the moment, Mr. Dunn bids adieu. He is courageous in a way few of us can measure let alone achieve.

I believe that the character of a man is reflected not by his actions in the light of day, but rather by those in the shadows of the night. I also believe that a man's character is measured not by how he celebrates his conquests but rather by how he handles his defeats.

Six Letters - Part 3

Hello Doc.
I'm feeling pretty rough.

I believe this here fighter has fought his last round.
The judges signal over and mark me down.
Sometimes, one's dealt a pretty bad hand.

Now one can simply bitch and whine, or
Pull close the cards and play on.

Let all know if they choose to ask,
That though I lost, I never folded.

Thanks Doc.

Voice Over
"Mr. Wilson, It is a pleasure to see you today. Let us catch up."

&

He speaks haltingly- not only because the stroke has affected his ability to enunciate but also because he has been profoundly affected by the tragedy. A lesson learned too late but learned nonetheless.

&&

Patients teach us constantly. Little do they realize how much their struggles force us also to re-evaluate our priorities.

Busy Man - Part 3

I'm sorry I'm late, but after a stroke, one doesn't walk quite as fast.

Doc,
I realize you had a point.
Absent health -
Of what value are riches?
To what end is power?

Oh, the cupcake?
My secretary reminded me -today I'm 47.
Surely you have time to celebrate and share?

Voice Over
"Mr. Vincent, It has been awhile since we last crossed paths."

&

He begins his story with an air of macho bravado but soon becomes pensive, thoughtful and slightly bewildered. He ends with a stunning admission of fear.

&&

Sometimes what a man finds most disconcerting is not his confrontation with Evil, but rather his encounter with Good.

Angels

Doc, do you believe in angels?

You realize I am a Marine.
I've fought in Hell and never flinched.
I've spit in the face of Death and dared her to strike.

Yet something very curious and so strange occurred - I need to share.

Six months ago, my heart began to fail and soon I found myself
Strapped to a cart and waiting for the surgeon's knife.
Have you ever been in the O.R. holding room?

The lights are blinding and blazing hot.
And the noise - Oh God!
The beeps, the buzzers, the alarms - constant and discordant.
The voices - soft and distant - the muffled cries of the injured and the ill.
The cacophony is incomprehensible.

"Hello Mr. Vincent.
I'm Dr. Arnold and I'll be putting you to sleep. Do you have any allergies?
Hello Mr. Vincent
I'm Nurse Akers and I'll be putting in a venous line.
Hello Mr. Vincent
I'm Nurse Davidson and I'll be putting in a second venous line.
Hello Mr. Vincent
I'm Nurse Thompson and I'll be putting in a catheter.
Hello Mr. Vincent
I'm Dr. Billings and I'll be putting in an arterial line.

Now what surgery are you having today?
Who is your doctor?
Have you said good-bye to your wife?"

Panic seized me - an icy grip closed tightly upon my throat.
My breath came fast - hard - and sweat burned my eyes.
I prayed to God.

And then the orderly who wheeled me in came back again.
Brought her face within six inches of mine, and said
"Now Mr. Vincent, everything will be alright - have no fear."

And the darkness of anesthesia blotted out all consciousness.

You realize I'm a Marine.
I've marched to Hell and never stumbled.
I've laughed in the face of Death and then turned my back upon her.

But one month ago, I met an angel and I am so afraid.

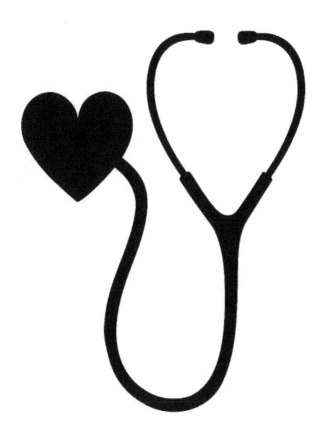

Voice Over

"Mr. Richards, you are in a fine mood today."

Pure unadulterated pride in a task done very well.

There are encounters so entertaining that you almost feel obligated to pay the patient for his performance. When he leaves the office, you can only shake your head and recite an old German proverb - "Gott hat eine grosse tiergarten" (God has a great zoo).

Blood Pressure

I've finished Doc!
You know when you ask an engineer to do a project,
he doesn't miss an angle.
Blood pressure 3 times a day for two months.

By date, by time, by position,
Even by side and size of cuff.

I have calculated mean and measured mode,
Squared the sum of the diastolics and added ten.

Regression analysis of systolics by even and odd days.

This chart shows blood pressure by activity –
Why the blip? Lady Vols were in a nailbiter.

And have correlated values with phases of the moon.

Pretty impressive huh?

Voice Over

"Mr. Jeffers, you seem very quiet today."

Metaphorically, he has come to a crossroads, and he must now choose a path. He understands, and that is what makes him so anxious and pensive, that there is no turning back. He crosses the Rubicon.

Faith and trust are two of the most inexplicable and powerful emotions. To prove or disprove another's disposition towards you, cataloguing behavior is a futile exercise. Why? For the same evidence can be interpreted with opposite valences.

Example: A smile and a kiss. Is this to throw one "off the track" or a sign of deep affection? Depends on whether you trust them or not.

A Point in Time

There comes a moment - a point in time
When all reasoned thought must cease.

Is she now faithful or will she once more stray?
Does she speak the truth or does she lie?
Does she truly understand or is it still a game?

One cannot mold another person's life nor bend their thoughts.
The path they take is theirs to choose.

One can only walk and pray she walks beside.

Voice Over

"Dan, you look lost in thought. Can I help?"

He is bewildered, confused, and cognizant of his error. The truth is awful, and the clock cannot be rewound.

Freud got it right even if he did not know where the amygdale lay. Primal forces of anger and desire drive our actions towards ends we fear. The rabbis say: "Who is strong? He who controls his passions."

Lost

What brought me to this point? I wish I knew.
There are forces whose currents run far beneath the surface of our
consciousness.
Beyond the reach of rational thought.
Yet, nonetheless compel a man to swim a course against his better nature.
The dictates of reality wage war against our fantasies.
But all too often, when we finally have seized our dreams, We grasp a
nightmare.

Voice Over

"Mrs. Ratle -what brings us together today?"

Peevish, irritated, impatient, and very unhappy. No matter how hard one tries to listen, she senses that you wish she were not there.

Patients of this sort constitute a challenge on many levels. It is very easy to dismiss them as somatizing, self-centered fools. Yet you know that serious illness can nonetheless lurk within their bodies. So what tests to order? Their deep rooted malaise infects one's own spirit. Her sadness beckons for understanding.

Questions

I'm so tired - don't tell me to lose weight, that is not the answer.
Anyway, I eat like a bird so it must be my thyroid.

When I bend forward, my back hurts.
When I walk, my legs ache.
When I reach to turn off the fan, my shoulders burn.
Do you think I have "fibro"?

There is this funny spot on my leg- I think it's cancer - take it off today!

I burn when I pee and I have lots of mucus when I poop.

Sex is no fun - hurts you know where.

When I eat, I get nauseated and my stomach swells.
You said taking out the gallbladder would help.

Doc, are you listening to me or are you going to act like my husband?

Voice Over

"Mrs. Holston, is there any way I can help?"

Anger and sadness hold sway in this woman's soul. She fears nothing at this point - even confrontation with the Almighty!

⅋⅋

A child's failures weigh so heavily upon parents' minds. They search their memories for clues as to why they erred. We are so mechanistic in our reasoning - for every action there has to be a cause. And so legalistic - someone must be at fault, if things go awry. Bad luck, not much to fall back upon to salvage peace of mind.

A Good Kid

He got five years in the penitentiary!
How could he have strayed so far?
Why did he stray?
He was such a good kid.

He lacked for nothing - clothes, money, vacations.
To the best schools he went.
I never missed a game and drove him everywhere
He wished to go.

It's in the genes? Is that what you say?
So I'm half at fault and my husband equally so.
Or does one of us bear full responsibility for his sorry state?

You don't know and never will.

How 'bout bad luck?
Wrong friend, wrong place, wrong time?
And let me "duke" it out with God.

Voice Over

"Mrs. Rice - Hello."

&

She encounters in her son an enigma that cannot be understood. And so without emotion, she simply describes.

&&

How little of the mind do we understand? Just ask those who study schizophrenia. It is impossible to comprehend the confusion and absolute chaos that reigns supreme in such a person's mind.

Schizophrenia

He rocks motionless, uncertain of the time.
Thoughts crowd his consciousness, obscuring reason.

Fiction or perhaps ancient fact molded into modern myth
Compel him to wrestle with demons never seen
Or sing with angels, voices distant.

His world spins in a universe beyond our ken,
Our paths cross yet never meet.

He rocks motionless, uncertain of the time.

Voice Over

"William, you look beyond fatigued. What is the matter?"

He is a desperate man. Deprived of restful sleep, agitated by thoughts seemingly not of his own making, he has literally reached the point of no return.

&&

OCD can drive a man to the brink and even over. We marvel at the mind's capacity to endure the most horrific assaults and lament its ability to self-destruct. Which pathways in our brains give us strength and which lead us into the darkest of woods?

Obsession

My thoughts pursue me as wolves maddened by the frenzy of the chase.
The scent of blood wafts through their nostrils, intoxicating them For they know their quarry falters.

I wheel, parry and thrust.
But they retreat, howling derisively, beyond the reach of my futile flailings.

I seek refuge in the dark of night but they seize my dreams and I awaken exhausted.

O God!
Heed my distress!
End this hunt - or I shall!

Voice Over

"Cynthia, you look too tired to speak but your face tells much."

In a monotone that is even more frightening because of the content of her words, Cynthia contemplates her end.

It is awful to watch a person slip into the clutches of depression - akin to witnessing the slow submersion in a pond of quicksand. You know that without action, tragedy is inevitable. The disease itself renders the victim unwilling to act on their behalf. A train wreck in slow motion with very little noise until the final crash.

Exit - Stage Left

I feel so bad.
It is as if a cold wet gray mist has wrapped itself around the world
Banishing all light and warmth from every nook and cranny.

Sleep, once my refuge and closest friend is now foe - fearsome and frightful.
- Food has no taste.
Nothing gives me pleasure.
Voices grate.
How dare you in my presence laugh?

So how is my world?
Children?- growing nicely.
Work? - no problems.
Husband? - he works so hard.
Every night he comes home late and every other weekend too.
I have never seen him travel so much.
I wish I had his ambition.
What am I?
Perhaps it would be best if from this boring play I took my leave.

Voice Over

"Mr. Jeffers - how are things fairing?"

⚬

Musing out loud is how he shares his thoughts; if the doctor wishes to listen in - fine.

⚬⚬

The more intimate a relationship, the more violent the conflict when it falls apart. And yet, if reconciliation is at all possible, reunion is extraordinarily tender.

Reconciliation

We are like two boxers who have bludgeoned themselves into
a state of utter exhaustion.
Too tired to raise a fist;
But unwilling to concede defeat,
We stand facing each other, unrecognizable, wondering how it will end.

Then, you raise your arm, not in defiance but
tentative, uncertain of my response.
I raise mine, they touch

We embrace and tears wash our wounds.

Voice Over
"Mrs. Rolston, you appear very upset. What can I do?"

&

She has a hard time controlling her emotions. First, seething anger towards her husband; then towards herself. And then a cry of anguish as she begs for understanding and mercy.

&&

When terrible things are done to us, we initially strike back at our assailant. But often, there follows a period of self recrimination as we try to uncover our faults, the ones that made him do it. Is this punishment for our sins; if so, for how long?

Retribution

Where should I start?
The beginning- is that what you said?

Came home last week with the groceries, slipped quietly in so as not to wake
My sleeping husband.

Then from the bedroom heard the sounds.
It has been a long time since I had sex, but one never forgets
The noises two people make.

He was with a girl whose laugh I initially did not recognize,
but then the squeal-
It was our daughter!

We keep a gun by the kitchen table and I reached, determined to destroy
what had Just destroyed me.
But upon the table sits a Bible and upon its
open page I read Christ's challenge:
"Let he who has not sinned, cast the first stone."
I never touched the gun.

Am I so evil?
What crime did I commit?
I never worked and never will.
Married a beast and sired two of the sorriest
excuses for adults the world has ever seen.
I've tried to be a good wife but I can't help the way I look.

My life is so empty -
No it isn't - it's like a cup overflowing with bitterness and despair.

How much pain must one endure before God lifts the press of thumb
And extends an open palm?

Voice Over

"Dan, what goes?"

This is a man lost and unable to envision any path out of the woods. He has come full circle. From boasting that he has it all under control, to whimpering for help.

&⁊&⁊

Actually, when one has hit rock bottom and feels totally lost, movement in any direction can be progress. He has yet to realize this. Not until he turns his focus from external signs will he begin the long slow climb from the bottom of the hole.

Direction

She has left me -
And now I stand at a crossroads whose sign lies buried in the leaves.

I cast a stone upon the earth to divine His plans –
If I turn left, what will Fate deliver?
If right, how will life unfold?

I scan the sky and listen to the winds for meaning and intent.
I count the clouds and cross my heart.

Then I turn to watch the trailing stranger,
He passes with nary a moment's pause.

I flip a coin - it stands on edge.

Voice Over

"Mr. Jeffers, I can tell you are a different man."

&

A quiet celebration. A rediscovery of what brings pleasure and what therefore truly matters.

&&

In the end, we define our most meaningful relationships very simply- a commonality of interests, a shared set of goals and days of "puttering together."

A Good Day

It was a good day.

There was no high drama,
No operatic passion,
No sex that "rocked the rafters."

But simply idle chatter and mundane chores.

Pictures to be hung- dishes to be stowed.
"You clean a room, I'll choose another."
"I'll run to the store; please sweep the garage."

Dinner for two.

"What shall we do when we retire?"
"Is there sufficient money for our children's school?"

There was no high drama,
No operatic passion,
No sex that "rocked the rafters."
Yet, it was a very good day.

Voice Over

"Mr. Richards, I can tell that you have much on your mind today."

This man has undergone a conversion, from one faith to another. He realizes this and yet has a hard time comprehending how it came to pass.

&&

We struggle individually and collectively to reconcile contradictory assertions: that the world is subject to the actions of a single deity but that each one of us is an autonomous being. Mr. Richards, I believe, succeeds marvelously.

Fate

We need to talk Doc.
You know me well.

I'm an engineer - a man of science - a rationalist supreme.
I value precision more than art.
Exactitude is my mantra.

For every effect there is cause and if we fail to see such
We have stumbled in our search.

Religion is for weak-willed fuzzy minds which flinch
At the world's complexities and posit deus ex machina.

Each day I leave work at 1630 - rarely a minute earlier, never one later.
I have charted my journey home to meter's length
And know at 1700, I'll speed across the bridge at Largent's Bay.
Set your clock by my travels - I dare you to do better.

Three weeks ago, I left my office and found a flattened tire.
A friend helped me repair the hole and oft I sped.

I never crossed the bridge that night.
At 1700, a barge broken free from its moorings, crushed the central pillars
And fifteen souls plunged to their watery grave.

Now, tell me how this can be!
What o'er arching plan drives our fortunes?
Why do I live to read of other's demise?
If there is cause, show me reason.

"A kingdom for a nail!"
A king lost his life for want of nail and I live for
having One too many.

I know now that though we navigate alone the currents Of our lives, with
back and limbs bent hard to task,

The channels Doc,
The channels by another's hand are cut.

Voice Over

"Mrs. Thomas, how are you?"

She has come to terms albeit uneasily, with her loss. It required first, a recognition of her insignificance.

How does one explain the inexplicable? By demanding answers from the One who rules us all! But sometimes, as Job discovered, the answers induce more questions.

Forever Gone

I challenged God!
God! God!
Why so young - why now?

And He replied.
Did you stand by my side when I split the heavens and raised the mountains
From the seas?

Whose breath gives wing to eagle and song to sparrow?
Whose hands orchestrate the tides and brush aside the early morning mists?

Whose finger colors the rainbow and
Whose tears bring forth flowers from the sand?

Answer me, and then I will answer you.

Voice Over

"Mr. Lessing, my condolences. Were you there at the end?"

❦

He reports without emotion the end; were the slightest emotion to appear, floodgates would shatter.

❦❦

Sometimes, the greatest act of love is to destroy that which we consider most precious. To say good-bye to that we feared to lose. To turn our back on that from which we never wished to part.

Death

She lay alone.
The pinched face of death staring open-mouthed at the wall. Breathing with
long hesitant pauses a few gulps of mortal's air.

Her limbs lay motionless and cool, Slate-blue against the whitened sheets.

I touched - eyelids flickered
A turning off, so imperceptibly slow, That the moment when passed
unnoticed.

Home

(The physician walks through his back door into the kitchen) I'm home.

Voice Over
"Long day?"

(The physician replies and pours himself a glass of water) Long day.

Voice Over
"Don't you get tired of hearing the same story day after day?"

(The physician takes a drink, raises the glass and replies) No - no I don't.

The End

CPSIA information can be obtained
at www.ICGtesting.com
Printed in the USA
JSHW040021090523
41439JS00002B/4